How to Effectively Treat Peripheral Neuropathy

INTRODUCTION

I want to thank you and congratulate you for downloading the book, " *The Neuropathy Cure* " .

Diabetic neuropathy means nerve damage caused due to diabetes, and it is one of the commonest causes of neuropathy known to us. One of many complications we associate with diabetes, Diabetic Peripheral Neuropathy (henceforth referred to as DPN) affects almost 60 % of diabetics at some point in time. A progressive disease, it results in loss of sensation, pain and weakness in the feet and sometimes, in your hands as well. DPN is more prevalent in people who find it difficult to manage their blood sugar levels.

The first thing that hits a person with DPN is numbness, pain or tingling in one's feet, legs or sometimes, hands. In the long term, it leads to a loss of reflexes and muscle weakness in the feet, specifically around the ankle region. With increasing nerve damage, loss of sensation in one's feet can reduce his/her ability to notice pain or to detect temperature. Since a person is unable to feel the pain caused by any injury to his feet, people with diabetic neuropathy often come to know of injuries, burns, lesions, etc only when they see it, which is often too late. Infections, sores and different types of outward damage to the foot is common in DPN patients.

Neuropathy caused by diabetes slowly progresses over time. It also can interfere with the normal functioning of the digestive system and sexual organs. 60% to 70% people who have had diabetes for long are affected by DPN.

How do you know if you have diabetic peripheral neuropathy? Make a note in case you are experiencing one or more symptoms from the list below. If your symptoms are in line with any in the list below, rush to your doctor.

If my feet tingle.
If you feel pinpricks in your feet.
If you have burning, stabbing and sometimes shooting pains in your feet.
If your feet are too sensitive to touch. For instance, sometimes it hurts when the bed covers touch your feet.
When sometimes you feel like you have socks or gloves on when you don't actually.
Your feet hurt at night.
Your feet and hands get extremely hot or extremely cold at times.

Your feet sometimes feel numb and dead.
You don't feel any pain, even though you have blisters or injuries on your feet.
You cannot feel your feet when you are walking.
The muscles in your feet and legs start becoming weaker with evert passing month and year.
If you start becoming unsteady when you walk or stand.
If you have trouble feeling heat or cold in your hands or feet.
When it seems like the muscles or bones in your feet have changed in shape.
When you have open sores or ulcers in your feet that heal very slowly.

Thanks again for downloading this book, I hope you enjoy it!

CHAPTER 1: ABOUT DIABETIC PERIPHERAL NEUROPATHY

Peripheral Neuropathy is a painful and debilitating condition caused due to some damage to the peripheral nervous system, or the complex network of nerves, which connect the central nervous system (the spinal cord and the brain) to the rest of the body. An estimated 25 million Americans are suffering from Peripheral Neuropathy, and a staggering 17 million of them (roughly 70%) are diabetics.

Diabetic Peripheral Neuropathy is a group of nerve disorders that are directly caused due to complications related to diabetes. Diabetic Peripheral Neuropathy may strike at any age, regardless of gender, age, or, for that any racial or ethnic background. People with diabetes who have trouble controlling their blood sugar levels, high blood pressure, high cholesterol, and obesity face an increased risk for developing DPN. It is the most common type of PN, and results in pain or loss of sensation in the legs, feet, hands and arms. This can lead to permanent damage to your body, along with a loss of sensation as well as ulcers, sores, and sometimes, lower-limb amputation. The longer you live with diabetes, the more are the chances of developing neuropathies, and people who have been living with diabetes for more than 25 years almost always suffer from DPN.

What are the reasons behind this damage to the nerves? Let us take a look at the possibilities.

Metabolic factors like high blood sugar, long history of diabetes, abnormally high blood fat levels, and low levels of insulin – all due to diabetes
Neurovascular conditions leading to damage to the blood vessels carrying oxygen and nutrients to the nerves
Autoimmune issues causing inflammation in the nerves
Mechanical nerve injuries, such as carpal tunnel syndrome (CTS)
Inherited nerve diseases
Lifestyle issues like smoking or alcohol use, etc.

Some of the symptoms of DPS are:

Numbness, tingling or a sensation of pain in the feet, toes, hands, legs, arms, and fingers

Damage of the feet or hand muscles
Sharp cramps or pains
Tremendous sensitivity to touch
Loss of coordination and balance
Weakness
Dizziness and fainting because of a drop in blood pressure
Stomach upset, diarrhoea or constipation
Hypoglycaemia, and an increasing tendency of failing to notice symptoms of low blood sugar
Erectile dysfunction
Difficulty urinating, etc.

Symptoms vary from patient to patient and may include abnormalities in the motor, sensory and autonomic—or involuntary—nervous systems. The first symptoms are, most often tingling, numbness or (mild or severe) pain in the feet. Sometimes, mild symptoms might go unnoticed for years in the beginning and increase in severity over the years. Sometimes, the onset of pain may be severe and sudden.

Though not directly associated with DPN, some people also experience depression. DPN can often lead to the loss of reflexes, especially at the ankle, and cause changes to the way that you walk. Foot deformities, like midfoot collapse, and hammertoe can occur. Again sores and blisters may develop in the foot that may be numb to the pressure or injury. Foot injuries, if not attended to, can cause infection deep into the bone and result in amputation.

How is DPN treated?

The first thing to do is to manage the levels of your blood glucose, and thus prevent further nerve damage. Managing your diabetes plays a critical role in treating DPN, so try to keep the blood sugar levels in normal range with proper diet, frequent testing, physical activity, diabetes medicine and/or insulin therapy. Most treatments for DPN are centered on pain reduction and improvement in function. Effective treatment for injured nerves often requires a combination of exercise, medicines and other therapies. It might take some time to arrive at the right combination for some. Medicines like ibuprofen and acetaminophen can sometimes effectively treat mild pain.

Common medicines prescribed are neuropathic pain agents, anti-seizure medicines or certain antidepressants.

Some medications used to help relieve diabetic nerve pain include:
Tricyclic antidepressants, such as Elavil or Cymbalta
Anticonvulsants, such as pregabalin (Lyrica), gabapentin (Gabarone, Neurontin)
Treatments that are applied to the skin-typically to the feet—include capsaicin
cream and lidocaine patches.
Important: Take excellent care of your foot. Studies indicate that nitrate patches or sprays for the feet may relieve pain. Alphalipoic acid, an antioxidant, and evening primrose oil have been known to relieve symptoms and may sometimes improve nerve function. Of course, do ask your doctor before using these. Supportive equipments include a device called a bed cradle that prevents bed-sheets and blankets from touching the sensitive feet and legs, physical therapy to increase strength of muscles, mobility and function, and also, orthopedic inserts or a specially designed shoe to even out improper gait. Treatments like magnetic therapy, electrical nerve stimulation and laser or light therapies are helpful. Take good care of your feet. Inspect your feet daily for blisters, injuries or sores, and wash carefully. Wear shoes or slippers to protect your feet, even when you're at home. Some insurance programs cover the costs of therapeutic shoes. If you need help with your care, see a podiatrist for advice and treatment.

Can eating right really help?

Diabetes is two kinds. Type 1 diabetes, or juvenile diabetes, is usually diagnosed at an early age and is the less common form of diabetes (cannot be prevented or reversed). Type 2 diabetes accounts for 90% to 95% of all diagnosed cases and most of them are preventable with timely healthy lifestyle changes. We have more control over your health than most of us believe. If you or your doctor is concerned about it, take control of your life —eat healthy, exercise regularly and keep your weight in check. Stick to a normal diet. Your nutritional needs are the same as everyone else. Proper eating habits can prevent and even reverse type 2 diabetes. Even if you already have type 2 diabetes, foods high in nutrients and low in fat, like vegetables, fruits and whole grains help you manage your condition effectively. Here are some other tips for eating right with diabetes on the next page.

What you eat: Making the right choices as far as your diet is concerned can make a big difference! Limit your refined carbohydrates and sugary drinks. For instance, drink skim milk instead of 2% or whole milk, choose water over soda, choose broiled or baked foods over fried, and try to limit daily sodium intake to no more than 2300 mg. Not sure where to start? Keep a food journal and discuss with your doctor about where you can improve.

When you eat: You are what you eat, but when you eat is just as important. Regularize your meal and snack timings to ensure consistency in blood sugar levels.

How much you eat: Size does matter. Even if you eat healthy, eating too much will promote weight gain, thus complicating your condition. Drinking lots of water is important to being healthy. Drink at least 2 liters of water each day. Eat foods with high water contents, like fruits.

Causes of peripheral neuropathy

There might be a various reasons that are responsible for causing peripheral neuropathy. It has been observed that those who have a family history of peripheral neuropathy tend to be more likely to develop this disorder. However, there are other factors and various underlying conditions, which might be responsible for causing this disorder. Following are the possible causes for peripheral neuropathy:

Generalized diseases

One of the most common forms of neuropathy is the nerve damage, which has been caused because of diabetes. A person suffering from this would experience numbness, pain and loss of sensation in their extremities. According to a study that was conducted by the University of Chicago's Centre for Peripheral Neuropathy, it was found that almost 60% of people who are suffering from diabetes will also have nerve damage in one form or the other. This damage is usually caused because of the high levels of blood sugar, and it was also found that amongst individuals who are diabetic, the risk of them suffering from neuropathy would increase if their blood sugar levels are high, they are overweight or they are above the age of 40 years.

There are some other major diseases, which are responsible for causing nerve damage is as follows:

Kidney failure and various other related conditions in which there is a buildup of a high level of toxins in the body can also result in considerable damage to the nerve tissue

When the body does not produce sufficient level of the thyroid hormone, this condition is known as hypothyroidism and when this occurs, it leads to retention of fluid and this would stress and pressurize the nerves surrounding this area.

Any disease that can cause severe inflammation, have the ability to spread to the nearby nerves and cause damage to the nerves as well as the connecting tissue surrounding the area affected.

There are certain vitamins that are essential to ensure nerve health and their functioning. And when a deficiency of vitamins like vitamin E, B1, B6 and B12 occurs, even this might cause neuropathy.

Any injury

One of the most common causes for injury to the nerves is physical trauma. And anything ranging from being involved in a car accident to a fracture might be enough to cause nerve damage. It is not just the happening of an event that might cause neuropathy but even prolonged periods of inactivity or even holding still for too long in one position might cause nerve damage. One of the most common types of neuropathy is carpal tunnel syndrome and it is caused when there is an increase in the pressure on the median nerve, this is a nerve that is responsible for supplying and facilitating movement and feeling in the wrist.

Alcohol

It is known that alcohol can cause damage to the nerves because the toxins in it will affect the nerve tissue. And people who suffer from alcoholism have a higher risk of contracting peripheral neuropathy. It is not just alcoholism but even exposure to certain toxic chemicals like insecticides, glue or even solvents; either voluntarily in the form of chemical abuse or in an involuntary form can cause severe nerve damage. Added to this there is another reason, exposure to mercury, lead or any other heavy metals can also be responsible for causing this condition.

Autoimmune disorders

There are certain viruses and bacteria that directly affect the nerve tissue. Some examples of such viruses would be herpes simplex or even the virus responsible for causing chicken pox and so on can cause some damage to the sensory nerves and it can also be responsible for the pangs of shooting pains an individual might experience. Infections caused by bacteria, such as Lyme disease can also be responsible for causing severe nerve damage and even pain if left untreated. Individuals who have HIV/AIDS are also susceptible to peripheral nerve damage. There are certain autoimmune diseases such a rheumatoid arthritis and even lupus; these affect the peripheral nerves and the peripheral nervous system in different ways. Severe or chronic inflammation and damage caused to tissues throughout your body, and even the pressure caused due to the inflammation can also be responsible for causing nerve pain in your extremities.

Medication

Medication given for fighting one condition might affect your body in some other way. Certain medications have the ability to cause nerve damage. For instance, drugs used to treat seizures, bacterial infections, medications used for treating cancer and even some medicines prescribed for even blood pressure have the ability to cause nerve damage. Recent research in this field of study has also shown that it is possible for statnis (drug used to reduce cholesterol and also helpful in prevention of cardiovascular disease) might also be able to cause nerve damage and also increase the risk of neuropathy.

CHAPTER 2: TYPES OF DIABETIC NEUROPATHY

Diabetic neuropathy can be classified into various categories. As you know, the human body comprises of various nerves and each of these nerves is associated with a different function of the body. Each of these neuropathies negatively affects these nerves. The symptoms of these neuropathies are different and the kind of treatment given depends upon the type of neuropathy. Diabetic neuropathy can be classified into four types and these are peripheral neuropathy, proximal neuropathy, autonomic neuropathy and focal neuropathy. More information about these types of neuropathy is provided below.

- **Peripheral neuropathy**

Peripheral diabetic neuropathy is also referred to as peripheral diabetic nerve pain and distal polyneuropathy. For a layman this might sound too complicated and elaborate. Therefore, for your convenience we will refer to it as either peripheral diabetic neuropathy or peripheral neuropathy. Isn't this much simpler?

One of the most common types of neuropathy caused because of diabetes is peripheral neuropathy. The nerves, which lead to your extremities, like arms, legs, hands and feet are affected because of this type of neuropathy. Did you know that the nerves going to your feet are the longest link of nerves present in the body? These nerves branch out of the spinal cord in the region of your lower back, also referred to as the lumbar region, before they head downwards towards your legs and ultimately to your feet. It is due to this incredible length of these nerves, they tend to be soft targets for this type of neuropathy because of the fact that these nerves provide a wider target because of the area covered by them. The nerve damage caused by this neuropathy often manifests itself in the form of various foot problems that are associated with diabetes including infections, ulcers, and foot deformities.

The various symptoms related to peripheral neuropathy are excruciating pain, the feeling of numbness, tingling sensation, weakness of muscles, cramping or twitching of muscles, there have been cases of either extreme sensitivity towards even the slightest touch and also extreme insensitivity towards pain or temperature and all these symptoms just get worse with nightfall.

- **Proximal neuropathy**

Proximal neuropathy is also referred to as diabetic amyotrophy. When we split the word amyotrophy, the word myo in it means muscles. So the simplest understanding of this type of neuropathy is as the form of neuropathy, which affects the muscles, thereby causing muscle weakness, especially those muscles present in the upper part of your legs, hips and buttocks. At times proximal neuropathy also manifests itself in the form of nerve pain, and this pain usually stems out of the lower back and goes down the leg. The appropriate medical term for this condition is radiculopathy; it is also referred to as sciatica by most people. Polyradiculopathy-diabetic amyotrophy is the condition where this pain stemming from nerves is added to the above mentioned troubles. This is the second most widespread form of diabetic neuropathy after peripheral neuropathy. And this usually affects elderly people with diabetes. When compared with peripheral neuropathy, it is possible to resolve proximal neuropathy. All it needs is time and treatment. The symptoms of proximal neuropathy such as weakness in the legs and also they have trouble while standing up without any help from a seated position. And usually this pain goes away after several months.

- **Autonomic neuropathy**

There are two types of functions that are performed by our body and these are voluntary functions and involuntary functions. The functions which are performed by our body consciously and involve thought process are known as voluntary functions and then there are certain functions performed by our body without you even thinking about them. Like the manner in which blood is pumped by your heart, breathing and also the way food is digested in your stomach. These actions take place, but you aren't conscious of their happening. Such functions are controlled by the autonomic system and it is also referred to as the autonomic nervous system. Then normal and well-balanced state of the human body is known as homeostasis and it is maintained by the autonomic nervous system. If there were any damage caused to any of the autonomic nerves because of diabetes (also known as autonomic diabetic neuropathy) then it would be difficult for the body to maintain homeostasis. But there is one important thing you should remember about autonomic neuropathy, the symptoms you exhibit would depend upon the damage caused to a specific nerve in the autonomic nervous system. This condition would seem extremely scary given that there are so many vital functions of the body, which can be damaged because of autonomic neuropathy.

If the nerves relating to the cardiovascular system were damaged then the symptoms would include irregular heart rate and dizziness or even fainting after standing. When the digestive system is affected the symptoms would include constipation, bloating, nausea, diarrhea and vomiting. When the optical nerves are affected then the person would experience trouble seeing clearly especially at night or when there is a sudden change in light, like when you step into sunlight from a dark building. The symptoms displayed when the reproductive system is affected would be in the form of erectile dysfunction for men and vaginal dryness in women. When the sweat glands are affected, the symptoms for autonomic neuropathy would be excessive sweating (especially after having certain types of food or during night time) and the other symptom would be reduction in sweating especially in the legs and feet. Bladder dysfunction is caused when the nerves in the urinary system are affected.

Because of nerve damage there is another condition, which might be caused, and it is known as hypoglycemia unawareness, this occurs when the responses, which are usually generated by our body when the blood sugar is low don't kick in due to the nerve damage. This condition is extremely dangerous for people who are suffering with diabetes, because they wouldn't be aware how and when their blood sugar level drops down. According to the damage to the autonomic nerves and the corresponding functions they control, the symptoms will vary.

- **Focal neuropathy**

The above-mentioned types of diabetic neuropathy, be it peripheral, autonomic or even proximal neuropathy are all examples of polyneuropathy. In polyneuropathy multiple nerves are affected. In contrast to this, in focal neuropathy only one specific nerve will be affected, and hence the name focused neuropathy. This condition is also referred to as mononeuropathy. The nerves in the head, especially the optic nerves are affected by focal neuropathy and it comes on suddenly. It is not just restricted to the head; the nerves in the torso and legs can also be affected by focal neuropathy. Proximal neuropathy also affects legs, but when focal neuropathy affects legs the symptoms are different. Proximal neuropathy causes the muscles in the legs to weaken and also causes shooting pain your leg, whereas in focal neuropathy, pain is caused only in specific locations on the legs.

Like I have already mentioned earlier, focal neuropathy sprouts up suddenly and its symptoms are not long term and usually disappear after a couple of weeks. Some o the possible symptoms of focal neuropathy when the nerves in the head are affected would be trouble of vision (it can be in the form of double vision, pain behind the eye and difficulty in focusing) and sudden paralysis of the face on one side, also known as Bell's palsy. The symptoms displayed when the nerves in the torso are affected are pain in the chest, lower back, stomach and the side. And lastly when the nerves in your legs are affected because of focal neuropathy the symptoms would include pain on the inside of the foot, shin and the front of the thigh.

CHAPTER 3: MORE ABOUT NEUROPATHY

Neuropathy need not be just sensory it can be motor or even autonomic. Each of these nerves is responsible for different functions performed by the human body. The sensory nerves are responsible for telling us how different things feel. The contraction of muscles and the initiation of movement are controlled by the motor nerves. The autonomic nerves are responsible for all the involuntary functions of the body like the beating of our heart, breathing, blinking of our eyes, and digestion of food and so on. The various symptoms exhibited would differ depending upon not just the location of the nerves but also the type of function performed by those nerves. Some of the most common symptoms are numbness, tingling sensation, pain and extreme weakness. Someone who is suffering from neuropathy would notice these symptoms and they would also notice that it is difficult for them to perform certain basic tasks like standing up, raising their arm over the head or even walking upon the stairs. These are normal tasks and yet they require more effort than necessary when the person is suffering from neuropathy.

Usually when you experience such symptoms, your doctor will refer to a neurologist. A neurologist is a doctor who not just specializes in the diagnosis of nerve and nervous system disorders but will also provide the necessary treatment to fight it. For the neurologist to decide the right course of action to help you fight neuropathy there are certain tests, which would need to be conducted before the treatment can begin. Like I have already mentioned there are various things which can cause neuropathy and this chapter and the coming chapters will talk about the various types of neuropathies, their symptoms and also the treatment options which are available. It is important to understand that there each neuropathy displays different symptoms, but it is not always necessary. More than one type of neuropathy can display similar symptoms. Therefore it is very important to make the right diagnosis so that the correct form of treatment can be adopted. When you visit a neurologist, please make sure that you have disclosed even the smallest of details. It might seem unrelated to you, but might in fact be related to the neuropathy you are suffering from. Be honest and disclose all the details.

Neurological exam
The thought of getting a complete neurological exam might scare you. But don't worry. It is not a scary procedure and it will help you before hand to

know all the various steps included in it. This way not only will you be aware of all the necessary bases your neurologist must cover but will also ensure that you are in the loop. So let us take a look at various steps, which are included in a complete neurological exam.

- ***Complete history of health***

The first and the most important step is that your neurologist should have the data about your complete health record. It is essential that your neurologist should spend time understanding the history of symptoms displayed by you, including the type of the symptoms, the duration for which they occur, the location and their onset. Such specific details about the reasons for the occurrence of these symptoms, the sensations caused by them and what relives these will help the neurologist arrive at a diagnosis, which is definite.

- ***Neurological evaluation***

Once the neurologist has obtained the history of your symptoms, the next step would be to conduct a physical examination to test your reflexes, strength and your ability to feel various sensations, in addition to a thorough evaluation of your autonomic nerves. This helps in reaching an overall diagnosis.

- ***Blood test***

Blood tests are very common and extremely essential to help with diagnosis. The neurologist would order some blood tests to check for any vitamin deficiencies present, blood sugar level, presence of infections, functioning of the immune system and the presence of toxins.

- ***EMG***

EMG stands for electromyography. This is the process of electrically measuring and recording the activity of various muscles. If there is any damage to any muscle, nerve or neuromuscular joint, all this will be revealed in an EMG. The neurologist would get to know the location of damage, if any.

- ***Nerve conduction studies***

This test helps in finding the damage caused to the peripheral nervous by measuring the speed and the efficiency of the electrical signals transmitted by these nerves. If there is any abnormality in this, then the neurologist will be able to identify it. Nerve conduction study and an EMG would go hand in hand.

- ***MRI***

MRI stands for Magnetic Resonance Imaging and it might be conducted as a rule, to rule out or eliminate any other causes of the neuropathy, like trauma, impingement or so on.

- ***Lumbar puncture***

A lumbar puncture is also known as spinal tap and it is usually performed to look for the presence of a protein or anything else in the spinal fluid, which would be the probable cause of neuropathy.

- ***Biopsy***

The last step would be to conduct a nerve or muscle biopsy. For doing this, a small piece of the muscle or the concerned nerve might be taken in order to figure out the cause for damage. But these tests are done only when there are certain specific conditions and symptoms or else it can be used as a method of elimination to rule out any possible cause.

Idiopathic neuropathy

A disease or a condition is said to be idiopathic when the cause or its origin is not known. This is the most common type of neuropathy found and it makes for about one third of all the neuropathic cases. To put it simply, this diagnosis means that the cause of the neuropathy is not known. The symptoms of idiopathic neuropathy are tingling sensation, numbness and a shooting pain which starts at the shins and also the balance of a person while walking or standing will also be affected because of this condition, added to this another symptom would be severe cramping of the muscles. Like stated earlier the neurologist will have to perform all the required tests, which will help him, either rule out the other possible causes or helps him identify it as idiopathic neuropathy. When either of these is done, only then can the plan of action to deal with this condition can be formulated and the treatment can start.

But then again, all this is dependent upon not just the location but also the type of nerves, which have been affected. Treatment for idiopathic neuropathy would consist of taking safety precautions to deal with the balance issues and also the loss of sensation, the other route, which can be adopted, is by using over the counter pain medication.

Diabetic neuropathy

When a person who has diabetes mellitus also has blood sugar levels which are above the normal one, might be one probable cause for why diabetic neuropathy might occur. The nerve fibers can slowly get damaged due to the presence of excess sugar in the blood stream. Because there isn't just one nerve which can get affected, any nerve present in the body can get affected and the symptoms can vary and they include constipation, dizziness, impotency, bladder problems, uncomfortably painful feet, indigestion and even some numbness in the feet. The tests which can be conducted would include EMG and nerve conduction study added to a complete blood work up to check for the glucose levels and a thorough neurological assessment of the individual. It is quintessential that the neurologist does a thorough assessment to identify the cause of neuropathy. It is important to understand the cause so that the proper treatment and course of action can be adopted and also to avoid improper assumptions such as high levels of sugar in a diabetic individual might not be the reason for the neuropathy. The treatment depends upon the area affected and the nerves damaged and also the symptoms experienced by the individual. Following a strict diet and complying with the diabetes medication will help maintain the required level of blood sugar and this is the first step of the treatment process. The next step is to take precautions to ensure that the existing problem doesn't worsen and it does not recur. What can be done further is to follow a strict diet and to take proper foot care, taking the necessary medical treatment for indigestion and constipation, prescribed antibiotics for relieving the bladder infection and reducing the pain.

Hereditary neuropathy

Something that is passed on through genes is known as hereditary and like the name suggests hereditary neuropathy is inherited through genes without any knowledge of it. For instance conditions like Charco-Marie-Tooth Disease and Pressure Palsies are hereditary. A disorder that is hereditary and affects two sets of nerves, both the motor and the sensory peripheral nerves is Charcot-Marie-Tooth disease. Symptoms of this disease are certain deformities in the feet or legs and these symptoms start showing up during the adolescent years and also the early stages of mid-adulthood. There are different types of CMT and the progression of this disorder is quite slow. This disorder is nothing but a mutation of the genes that are responsible for the structure of myelin sheath and/or the peripheral nerve axon. And all these ultimately have an effect on the communication between the brain and the muscles. This disorder would cause severe deformities of the legs and therefore one therapeutic measure would be the use of leg braces, other options are physical therapy or occupational therapy and also the use of such devices that would help with improving the deformities and also assist in improving upon them to. When hereditary neuropathy has been combined with Liability to Pressure Palsies is a hereditary neuromuscular disorder and when someone is suffering from this disorder it would make them soft targets for damage to their nerves due to repetitive movements or compression. This resultant pressure, though it is very minimal would result in increasing insensitivity or even weakness in the limb that has been affected. This state usually lasts longer and the person suffering from this disorder would experience the feeling of his or her leg "falling asleep" but for a longer duration. Carpal tunnel syndrome would be the resultant injury. Therefore, to be in the clear it would be safe for a person who is suffering from carpal tunnel syndrome to also get a complete check up done to ensure that it isn't hereditary neuropathy. For diagnosing hereditary neuropathy it would be necessary to give your neurologist a comprehensive and detailed medical history and a complete neurological exam, an EMG, nerve biopsy and genetic blood testing too. Over the counter medication will help the sufferer fight off the pain and ergonomic training will help reduce or avoid any injuries which might arise out of daily activities.

- **Immune neuropathy**

There are various types of immune or inflammatory neuropathies, and these neuropathies are extremely rare and would require a thorough checkup for it to be discovered. Amongst these neuropathies, there are two disorders that are most common and these are Multifocal Motor Neuropathy and Chronic Inflammatory Demyelinating Polyneuropathy. The former disorder mentioned (Multifocal Motor Neuropathy) is characterized by general weakness and the degeneration of the muscles related to hands and ankles, but this isn't always the case as it can affect other muscles too. It can be confusing to diagnose this disorder because the weakness can be severe or just minimal in a few muscles or all the limbs. Such extreme scenarios presented by this disorder make it difficult to diagnose. Since it has an effect on only the strength of the muscle and not the sensation, in some cases it has been mistaken for Amyotrophic Lateral Sclerosis.

The latter (Chronic Inflammatory Demyelinating Polyneuropathy) is an autoimmune disease. An autoimmune disorder is a condition wherein the immune system of a person would attack itself, thereby causing extreme weakness and the person would also develop abnormalities related to senses and this would go on for a few months before stabilization can be achieved. Or for that matter it would take several months for the condition to improve and there might be relapses too. This disorder can affect people belonging to any age group and the severity of the condition can vary from mild to extremely severe. Though it usually is not painful, there have been cases where the patients express unusual or bothersome sensations in their hands and feet.

Both of the above mentioned conditions are caused when the immune system attacks the peripheral nerves present in the body. The myelin sheath is the protective layer covering the nerves and then there are certain ion channels present in our nerves and these channels help in passing on the electrical signals throughout the body. And these are the two aspects of the human body, which come under fire when the immune system attacks the peripheral nerves. When this happens, these electrical signals get disturbed and blocked causing them to stop moving and thereby the nerves get injured. These neuropathies are incredibly rare and quite difficult to diagnose. A neuromuscular disease specialist is someone who specializes in neuropathy and an opinion of such an expert would usually be required for identifying these neuropathies. Only an expert will be able to identify the presence of any unusual or odd sensory loss or muscle weakness and this can be identified only after conducting a comprehensive nerve conduction studies.

CHAPTER 4: TYPES, SYMPTOMS AND DIAGNOSIS OF DPN

More about peripheral neuropathy

Peripheral neuropathy, as it names suggests occurs when the peripheral nerves are damaged and it often causes weakness, severe pain and numbness in areas in and around feet and hands. But it isn't restricted to just these areas and any other part of the body might also be affected. The duty of a person's peripheral nervous system is to transmit the information processed by the brain to the rest of your body through your spinal column. The causes why a person might be suffering from peripheral neuropathy are varied. It can be a result of an inherited condition, problems related to metabolism, infections, exposure to toxins and even traumatic injuries. Though one of the most common reasons of why this disorder occurs is diabetes mellitus.

As you already know by now, the peripheral nerves are responsible for delivering and receiving the signals related to physical sensation to your brain and then the parts of the body concerned. This disorder occurs when the peripheral nerves or the nerves responsible for relaying this communication are damaged or malfunctioning, thereby disrupting or interrupting their usual activity. So what might happen is that these nerves might end up sending signals of pain when there is no reason as to why there should be any pain in the first place or they might not send a signal of pain even when something is in fact causing pain to the individual. People who are suffering from peripheral neuropathy often describe the pain borne by them as a stabbing or a burning sensation and there is tingling too. In many cases, the symptoms might improve, especially when an underlying disease that can be treated has caused it. Medication is also helpful to reduce the pain. Calling this disorder as uncomfortable is an understatement and treatments have been extremely helpful in many cases. But before the right course of action can be decided it is essential to determine whether this condition has been caused by an underlying condition which might be serious or not.

Types of DPN

The most common of all the diabetic neuropathies by far, DPN may be divided into two main categories (there are many other variants, but these are the major categories):

Acute sensory neuropathy or Hyperglycaemic neuropathy and
Chronic sensorimotor neuropathy also known as symmetric distal polyneuropathy

Acute sensory neuropathy is a type of symmetrical poly-neuropathy with an acute or sub acute onset characterized by severe sensory symptoms, usually with almost no clinical signs. It can be diagnosed by an episode of glycemic instability, and it gets better with better when you control your diabetes. Usually, complete recovery takes no more than 12 months. Proper control of diabetes is the key to get rid of sensory neuropathy and wild fluctuations may be associated with burning pain. Another thing to remember is that all DPN patients may experience a spike in pain at night. Movement of the area near the ankle may be affected and ankle reflexes suffer.

Chronic sensorimotor neuropathy is the most common type of DPN. It is usually seen in up to 50% of long suffering diabetes patients. Although almost half the DPN patients don't show any symptoms, 10–20% of sufferers experience distressing symptoms sufficient to warrant specific therapy. Sensorimotor neuropathy can sometimes be accompanied by autonomic dysfunction. It may lead to Charcot neuroarthropathy, foot ulceration and sometimes, amputation, (amputation should be preventable in most cases). Chronic DPN is caused by both age and duration of diabetes, and is more common when diabetes has not been controlled well. Chronic DPN most often affects the extremities of one's lower limbs, or the ankle downwards. Hands, calf muscles and areas above the knee are affected in only the most extreme cases. It may also lead to abnormal muscle sensory function, which manifests itself in unsteady movements. The vibration perception threshold is also affected.

What are the symptoms of peripheral neuropathy?

There are three types of peripheral nerves and each of these nerves affects a particular region of the human body. For instance, the sensory nerves are connected to your skin, the motor nerves are connected to your muscles and the autonomic nerves are connected to your internal organs. Peripheral neuropathy might affect any one or all the three of these nerves and therefore there isn't any particular part of the body this disorder might be constrained to. Every nerve, which is a part of the peripheral system, has got a certain specific role to play. And the symptoms that might exist will vary depending upon the type of nerve(s) that has been affected. As you already know, the nerves in this system are classified into three categories and these are:

- The nerves that facilitate in receiving sensation from skin, like temperature, pain, touch or even vibration, are known as sensory nerves.
- The nerves that are responsible for how you control your muscles are known as motor nerves.
- The nerves that are responsible for controlling function such as blood pressure, heart rate, digestion and all of the other involuntary functions are known as autonomic nerves.

When the peripheral nerves are affected, the symptoms which you might include the following:

- Pangs of sharp, burning or jabbing pain
- Numbness and/or tingling sensation that might gradually start from your hands and feet, this sensation might later on spread into your arms and legs
- You might experience extreme sensitivity towards touch.
- You might also experience the loss of coordination and take quite a few falls

When the motor nerves in your body are affected because of peripheral neuropathy, then there would be muscle weakness that might escalate to even paralysis.

When the autonomic nerves of the peripheral system that is responsible for controlling your involuntary functions have been affected, then you might experience the following symptoms:

- Developing intolerance towards heat and you might also experience altered sweating.
- Problems related to digestion, bowel movement or even the bladder
- Variations in the level of blood pressure might cause weakness,

dizziness and lightheadedness.

Peripheral neuropathy might be of three types and these are mononeuropathy, multiple mononeuropathy and polyneuropathy. In the case of mononeuropathy only one nerve might get affected, in the case of multiple mononeuropathy two or more nerves present in different areas will get affected and lastly, in the case of polyneuropathy multiple nerves might get affected.

For deciding the course of treatment the procedure followed will be similar to the one adapted for any of the neuropathies. Do not neglect any of these symptoms. And seek medical attention as soon as possible when you start noticing any unusual sensations like tingling, pain or even weakness in your hands and feet. The best chance you have got of controlling this disorder is early detection. Appropriate treatment will also help in controlling the damage done and will also preventing from any further damage to the peripheral nerves.

Therefore the first thing you need to do is consult your doctor as soon as you start noticing these symptoms. Don't withhold any of the details and explain all the symptoms you have been experiencing. The cause of the neuropathy will differ and according to it the course of treatment will also need to be modified.

Depending on the specific pattern of damage to nerve fibers of different size and function, the symptoms vary widely. A loss of sensation (like pain, touch, vibration, tingling, temperature, etc) and an inability to feel changes in temperature are usually the result of some damage to small sensory fibers of type C. Of course, there is a tendency to get sores in the feet and these sores do not heal as quickly as they should. Sometimes, it hurts even when a patient's foot comes in touch with the bed sheet.

Numbness is the most common symptom in patients of diabetic peripheral neuropathy. The inability to feel your feet while walking is a common occurrence. At other times, your hands or feet may tingle or you might feel a burning sensation. You may feel like as if you are wearing a glove or a sock even when you're not.

Often, the pain will be sudden and sharp, resembling an electrical current. You may also feel cramp when holding something like a piece of silverware.

Quite often, DPN sufferers tend to suddenly drop things due to the pain, numbness and loss of control.

Diabetic peripheral neuropathy patients often complain of a sudden lack of balance and walking with a wobbly motion. Wearing orthopaedic shoes might help in this situation. The most common sign of diabetic peripheral neuropathy is loss of coordination. Also, muscle weakness affects your ankle, which in turn affects your gait.

Deformities may show up in your foot. The main reasons behind this are the unusual shifts in weight make the patients walk abnormally. It happens due to loss of nerve function. DPN patients are often afflicted with hammertoe. (happens when one of the three toes lying between the big toe and the little one loses shape near the joint.)

You might suddenly notice blisters or sores on your feet that you can't explain. It happens when you hurt yourself and didn't feel it. That happens because the brain is unable to send a pain signal due to nerve damage. Hurting yourself and not noticing it can be extremely dangerous. Just imagine, what happens if you burn yourself with hot and not notice it due to numbness?

Exaggerated sensations is a common symptom of diabetic peripheral neuropathy. Holding a cup of even mildly warm coffee may become painful, and serious hurt can be caused when a person touches you with cold hands. Your hands or feet may feel hot or cold for no apparent reason.

DPN becomes more painful at night. You may hurt so much that a bed sheet feels extremely heavy and painful, making it difficult to sleep through the night.

Tips: Avoid tobacco and alcohol if you have diabetic peripheral neuropathy. These are known to worsen your suffering. Proper nutrition is extremely important, as vitamin deficiency encourages DPN. It can be managed effectively with proper medication. Unchecked wounds often lead to infections, so regularly check your arms and foot. In some cases, infections spread to the bone, which in turn could lead to amputation of toes and/or feet.

How to diagnose DPN?

When screening for DPN, usually a particular set of questions are asked to the patients. Examples of some typical questions are given below. The diagnosis should ideally be undertaken in the presence of a doctor, but the purpose of mentioning these questions in this book is to help the patient find (roughly) out if he/she suffers from DPN without going to a doctor. Of course, you would ultimately need to visit a doctor for treatment.

No. 1 Are your legs or feet numb?
No. 2 Do you ever experience any burning pain in your legs or feet?
No. 3 Are the feet overtly sensitive to touch?
No. 4 Do you occasionally get muscle cramps in your legs or feet?
No. 5 Do you ever feel that somebody is prickling in your legs or feet?
No. 6 Does it usually hurt when the bed covers come in contact with your skin?
No. 7 Are you able to distinguish hot water from the cold water with your feet?
No. 8 Did you ever have an open sore on your foot (most likely at the bottom of your foot)?
No. 9 Has your doctor ever told you that you have diabetic neuropathy?
No. 10 Do you feel experience a feeling of weakness often?
No. 11 Do the symptoms flare up at night?
No. 12 Do your legs usually hurt while walking?
No. 13 Are you able to sense your feet when you walk?
No. 14 Does the skin on your feet crack open due to dryness?
No. 15 Have you ever had an amputation?

Besides completing this questionnaire, the doctor needs to examine you (your feet and hands mainly) as well. Let us find out what are the things that a doctor usually checks. A doctor may ask for information about dry skin, other deformities, infection, callus, fissure, and others. They check for any abnormalities in extremities (like hands and feet), ulcers, and many other things.

Responses are added to obtain the total score. Responses of "yes" to questions 1-3, 5-6, 8-9, 11-12, 14-15 is each counted as one point. A "no response" on questions 7 and 13 is counted as 1 point. Question 4 (to measure any impairment in circulation) and question 10 are not included in the scores. A certain score might mean that you are affected, but as I said, Of course, you would ultimately need to visit a doctor for proper diagnosis and treatment.

Initial Therapy and Counselling

Once diagnosed, a doctor needs to give their patients a detailed explanation and set the right expectations about their condition, educate them and allay any fears or misconceptions. Letting them know that the pain would subside with some treatment and some time can be very reassuring. Simple physical treatments, such as the use of a bed cradle as discussed previously to lift the bedclothes off of hypersensitive skin may be helpful. Suitable footwear selection may also help and the doctor's advice plays an important role here. In patients with relatively mild symptoms, anti- inflammatory agents or analgesics may be effective enough.

Metabolic Control

The most effective way to achieving stable normalcy is pancreas or islet cell transplantation. However, this is not possible most of the times because it is only available to patients with end stage diabetic neuropathy who may opt for a combined pancreas and kidney transplants or in young people with type 1 diabetes. A number of recent studies suggest that stable sugar levels are of the greatest importance here. Recent studies assert that continuous glucose monitoring has confirmed that painful symptoms were indeed associated with inefficient diabetes control. Insulin therapy helps, of course, but there is no evidence that patients whose diabetes has been controlled effectively with oral hypoglycemic agents will get pain relief by switching over to insulin therapy.

Causes of peripheral neuropathy

There might be a various reasons that are responsible for causing peripheral neuropathy. It has been observed that those who have a family history of peripheral neuropathy tend to be more likely to develop this disorder. However, there are other factors and various underlying conditions that might be responsible for causing this disorder. Following are the possible causes for peripheral neuropathy:

Generalized diseases

One of the most common forms of neuropathy is the nerve damage that has been caused because of diabetes. A person suffering from this would experience numbness, pain and loss of sensation in their extremities. According to a study that was conducted by the University of Chicago's Centre for Peripheral Neuropathy, it was found that almost 60% of people who are suffering from diabetes will also have nerve damage in one form or the other. This damage is usually caused because of the high levels of blood sugar, and it was also found that amongst individuals who are diabetic, the risk of them suffering from neuropathy would increase if their blood sugar levels are high, they are overweight or they are above the age of 40 years. There are some other major diseases that are responsible for causing nerve damage is as follows:

Kidney failure and various other related conditions in which there is a buildup of a high level of toxins in the body can also result in considerable damage to the nerve tissue

When the body does not produce sufficient level of the thyroid hormone, this condition is known as hypothyroidism and when this occurs, it leads to retention of fluid and this would stress and pressurize the nerves surrounding this area.

Any disease that can cause severe inflammation, have the ability to spread to the nearby nerves and cause damage to the nerves as well as the connecting tissue surrounding the area affected.

There are certain vitamins that are essential to ensure nerve health and their functioning. And when a deficiency of vitamins like vitamin E, B1, B6 and B12 occurs, even this might cause neuropathy.

Any injury

One of the most common causes for injury to the nerves is physical trauma. And anything ranging from being involved in a car accident to a fracture might be enough to cause nerve damage. It is not just the happening of an event that might cause neuropathy but even prolonged periods of inactivity or even holding still for too long in one position might cause nerve damage. One of the most common types of neuropathy is carpal tunnel syndrome and it is caused when there is an increase in the pressure on the median nerve, this is a nerve that is responsible for supplying and facilitating movement and feeling in the wrist.

Alcohol

It is known that alcohol can cause damage to the nerves because the toxins in it will affect the nerve tissue. And people who suffer from alcoholism have a higher risk of contracting peripheral neuropathy. It is not just alcoholism but even exposure to certain toxic chemicals like insecticides, glue or even solvents; either voluntarily in the form of chemical abuse or in an involuntary form can cause severe nerve damage. Added to this there is another reason, exposure to mercury, lead or any other heavy metals can also be responsible for causing this condition.

Autoimmune disorders

There are certain viruses and bacteria that directly affect the nerve tissue. Some examples of such viruses would be herpes simplex or even the virus responsible for causing chicken pox and so on can cause some damage to the sensory nerves and it can also be responsible for the pangs of shooting pains an individual might experience. Infections caused by bacteria, such as Lyme disease can also be responsible for causing severe nerve damage and even pain if left untreated. Individuals who have HIV/AIDS are also susceptible to peripheral nerve damage. There are certain autoimmune diseases such a rheumatoid arthritis and even lupus; these affect the peripheral nerves and the peripheral nervous system in different ways. Severe or chronic inflammation and damage caused to tissues throughout your body, and even the pressure caused due to the inflammation can also be responsible for causing nerve pain in your extremities.

Medication

Medication given for fighting one condition might affect your body in some other way. Certain medications have the ability to cause nerve damage. For instance, drugs used to treat seizures, bacterial infections, medications used for treating cancer and even some medicines prescribed for even blood pressure have the ability to cause nerve damage. Recent research in this field of study has also shown that it is possible for statnis (drug used to reduce cholesterol and also helpful in prevention of cardiovascular disease) might also be able to cause nerve damage and also increase the risk of neuropathy.

Complication of peripheral neuropathy

There are certain complications that might arise due to peripheral neuropathy.

And since the peripheral nerves are more or less responsible for the well functioning of the body and also the control of all the vital organs and our sensory receptors too, when these nerves are damaged there will be certain complications that a person will have to face. These complications are as follows:

- When the nerves which transmit sensation from skin to brain and vice versa have been damaged then the individual will experience numbness and he/she might not feel any change in temperature or pain or the other possibility is that the likelihood of their sensitivity will increase. Whatever the case might be, the individual will have to face burns and skin trauma.
- When the peripheral nerves are damaged it is a very real possibility that you might lose sensation in certain parts of your body, especially your feet. So you might not even realize when you get hurt or injured. Therefore, to prevent any infection it is essential that you keep checking your feet and the other likely areas for any injuries and treat the ones found immediately to avoid infection. And if you have diabetes, then be doubly careful and keep checking for such injuries regularly.

Complication of peripheral neuropathy

There are certain complications that might arise due to peripheral neuropathy. And since the peripheral nerves are more or less responsible for the well functioning of the body and also the control of all the vital organs and our sensory receptors too, when these nerves are damaged there will be certain complications that a person will have to face. These complications are as follows:

- When the nerves which transmit sensation from skin to brain and vice versa have been damaged then the individual will experience numbness and he/she might not feel any change in temperature or pain or the other possibility is that the likelihood of their sensitivity will increase. Whatever the case might be, the individual will have to face burns and skin trauma.
- When the peripheral nerves are damaged it is a very real possibility that you might lose sensation in certain parts of your

body, especially your feet. So you might not even realize when you get hurt or injured. Therefore, to prevent any infection it is essential that you keep checking your feet and the other likely areas for any injuries and treat the ones found immediately to avoid infection. And if you have diabetes, then be doubly careful and keep checking for such injuries regularly.

CHAPTER 5: TREATING DPN

Visiting the doctor

As far as doctors for treating DPN are concerned, you might need to visit 3 kinds of doctors: endocrinologist, neurologist and a podiatrist. An endocrinologist is a doctor who specializes in dealing with metabolic issues like diabetes and other issues related to hormones. Remember insulin, which is critical to diabetes, is a hormone and an endocrinologist is critical to maintaining stable sugar levels. You may also need to visit a neurologist, a doctor that specializes in treating conditions related to nerves. The neurologist's role here is to diagnose the exact extent of damage to the nerves and suggest treatment specific to nerves. And finally, you may need to visit a podiatrist. A podiatrist is a foot doctor. Naturally, since most DPN patients face issues with the condition of their foot, visits to a podiatrist becomes essential sometimes.

Preparing for the appointment with your doctor

There is some amount of preparation needed before you visit the doctor the first time. You need to keep some information handy. Here are some of the questions that you may need to answer (possibly):

Ask the doctor or his/her staff if there are any pre-appointment restrictions. While make the appointment, ask how you need to prepare, like restricting your diet, etc.

Note down any important personal information, like any major stresses or any recent changes in lifestyle Jot down any symptoms you may be experiencing, and include all symptoms you are facing, even those that may seem unrelated to diabetic peripheral neuropathy. .

Write down your recent blood sugar levels. Taking daily readings for a week before the appointment.

Make a list of all medications, supplements and vitamins you have been taking of late or anything that you think may be related to your condition.

Take along a friend or a family member. It helps in case you forget to mention some essential details. Your doctor needs to know everything.

If possible, write down any questions you want to ask your doctor.

In fact, keeping a set of questions can help you best utilize the time with your doctor. Even if you don't have any questions right then, there are many questions that may occur to you in time and there is nothing better if you get your doctor to answer those for you. This also helps you know your condition better and take remedial steps. Here are some possible questions:

Would I need to undergo tests to confirm the diagnosis for my symptoms?
Would the tests require any specific preparations?
Is diabetes the root cause of my symptoms? How?
Would these symptoms disappear if I control my blood sugar effectively?
Is this going to be a temporary condition or a long term one?
What are the options available (for treatment), and which one would you recommend?
What if I have other health conditions? Would I be able to manage them together? If so, how?
What are the side effects I may possibly encounter in the course of the treatment?
Do you have any brochures or printed material I can read? What websites would you recommend to get more information about my condition?
Would I need to see other doctors, like a podiatrist or a dietician?

What are the questions a doctor might ask you?

Expect your doctor to ask you a number of questions. Here is a possible list for patients suspecting diabetic peripheral neuropathy:

How do you control your blood sugar?
Since how long have you been experiencing these symptoms?
Have you been continuously experiencing these symptoms or occasionally?
What is the level of severity of these symptoms?
What, if anything seem to give you relief?
What are the things that tend to aggravate your symptoms?
Which (if any) aspect of managing diabetes do you find most challenging?
How can you possibly manage your diabetes better?

Tests required for diagnosing diabetic peripheral neuropathy

To diagnosing diabetic peripheral neuropathy properly, your doctor would need to know the symptoms you face, your medical history and of course physical examination of your extremities. Some tests might need to be performed on you as well. Some of those tests are:

<u>Filament tests</u>, where your sensitivity to touch is tested with the help of a soft nylon fiber called a 'monofilament'. If you cannot feel the filament on your feet, it might lead the doctor to conclude that you have lost sensation in those feet nerves.

<u>Nerve conduction studies</u> that test how fast the nerves in your arms and feet conduct electrical signals. This test is also used to diagnose carpal tunnel syndrome, a condition of the wrist.

<u>Electromyography (EMG)</u> test that are usually performed with nerve conduction studies. Electromyography test measures the electrical discharges that your muscles produce.

<u>Quantitative sensory testing</u> is a non-invasive test often used to find out exactly how your nerves respond to changes in temperature and vibration.

<u>Autonomic testing</u> is done to find out if you have symptoms of autonomic neuropathy. This is a test that looks at your blood pressure in different positions and assesses your ability to sweat. Abnormal sweating is known to be a major symptom of diabetic peripheral neuropathy.

Principles of Treatment

We have already seen the various options of treatment available for treating peripheral neuropathy and the alternative medicines and therapies available to tackle this condition. There are two major goals of the treatment that is given for peripheral neuropathy. These goals are to control the process of the underlying disease and the second goal is to treat the bothersome symptoms. The first goal can be achieve by wiping clear all the troublesome agents and their residues, such as all the toxins or medications, rectifying the nutritional deficiency suffered by the person and also the treatment of the underlying disease (let us take the case of a neuropathy which is immune mediated, then this can be done in the form of corticosteroid therapy). These steps are important for not just halting the progress of the neuropathy but also this might help in improving the symptoms displayed because of this condition. But when it comes to acute inflammatory neuropathies, these will require a plan of action that is more quick and aggressive management by making the use of intravenous immunoglobulin or any of its substitutes. Just not this, but it is also recommended that there is a test done for respiratory functioning and also hemodynamic monitoring. When the vital capacity of the patient is below 20 ml per kg or if it has depreciated by an amount greater than 30% of the baseline, or the other scenario is when the maximum inspiratory pressure is less than 30 cm of water, then in any of these cases mechanical ventilation should be given a serious thought. Not just this, but it is also essential to facilitate the patients to get the difficult symptoms of peripheral neuropathy under control. These symptoms can vary from extreme pain and numbness. The other thing that needs to be kept in mind is to reduce the disability that might be resultant of the severe weakness suffered by the individual. There are various drugs available in the market, which will help alleviate pain, and they include antisiezure drugs, and antidepressants. In some patients it has also been found that topical patches and sprays, which contain lidocaine or capsaicin, will also help reduce or alleviate the pain they must be suffering. Other supportive measures should also be taken to increase the comfort and reduce the discomfort suffered by the individuals. These steps would be proving proper foot care, proper shoe selection and weight reduction too. Narcotics also have the ability to reduce the pain and therefore even they have found a place in the treatment of extreme neuropathic pain, but this must be applied to patients with caution. Before this option is considered it is essential to ensure that the candidates have been thoroughly screened for possible history or tendencies of substance abuse and addiction too. And this should be considered as the last resort. Before you move on to this, all the other non-narcotic options need to be considered and a second opinion in these cases can never hurt.

Treatments for peripheral neuropathy

Peripheral neuropathy occurs when the peripheral nerves in your body are damaged and there are different causes for peripheral neuropathy. Therefore the treatment you might use to deal with peripheral neuropathy will differ depending upon the area that has been affected and also the nerve that has been damaged. The first thing you need to do is consult your doctor and fix up an appointment with a neurologist to help you identify the cause of the neuropathy so that you can start with the treatment. There are many treatments available that will provide you relief and will also enable you to get back to your regular activities. At times it has proven to be beneficial to use a combination of treatments to deal with peripheral neuropathy.

- **Medications**

Medicines have always helped the individuals suffering from peripheral neuropathy in the battle against the disorder. The medication used can be prescribed medication or even over the counter medication. Both of these will help you with the pain. Medicines for relief from pain (pain killers) can be over the counter medicines, which can help relieve the mild symptoms, the drugs that contain no steroids and are anti-inflammatory, will help with this. This was in the case when the symptoms are mild. But when the symptoms are severe, then your doctor will give you certain prescribed pain relieving medications. There are certain medications, which consist opiods or oxycodone (drugs like oxycontin, Conzip and so on), but these medications need to be prescribed with caution. Because it might just so happen that the individual might get dependent on these and it might also lead to substance abuse. Therefore it is advisable that the doctor looks into the history of the patient for probable cause or reason for substance abuse. And these types of medications need to be used as the absolutely last resort. Consider this option when other treatments do not work, and not before that. Medication, which is usually prescribed to treat epilepsy, will also help reduce the nerve pain. Anti seizure drugs are often used to treat peripheral neuropathy. Though there are certain side effects of these drugs, therefore it is advisable that you thoroughly look into all the possible side effects before you start using these drugs.

There is a substance that is found in hot peppers which is known to relieve the pain. This substance is known as capsaicin. Though there might not be any drastic improvement in the symptoms of peripheral neuropathy once you start using any cream containing capsaicin, but you will find some moderate improvement. Doctors in combination with other treatments to ensure better results usually suggest this. Initially you might experience skin irritation or even burning sensations in the areas where you apply a capsaicin based cream. But with time these sensations will reduce gradually. But again, it all depends upon the capacity of tolerance exhibited by the individual. Because some people just cannot tolerate this substance. Antidepressant shave also been proven to be helpful in dealing with peripheral neuropathy. There are some specific tricyclic antidepressants like doxepin, notriptyline an dos on which have been proven to help reduce or relive the pain caused due to nerve damage by interfering with the chemical processes going on in your brain and spinal cord, and thereby reducing the pain because of disruption in the correspondence of signals which make you experience pain. These antidepressants help reduce the pain caused because of diabetes, but like any other medication even these have certain side effects. The side effects of using antidepressants include dryness of the mouth, sleeplessness, drowsiness, dizzying sensation, decrease in appetite and certain problems related to the digestive system like constipation and indigestion.

Your doctor might also prescribe certain medication that will help you deal with the underlying conditions that are the cause for peripheral neuropathy. There might be certain medication prescribed to help reduce the inflammation in your body, or even the aggressiveness of your immune system's reaction. This will help the individual deal with the autoimmune condition prevalent in order to control the peripheral neuropathy. Pain medications that you can get over the counter like Tylenol, and anti-inflammatory drugs such as aspirin and ibuprofen will also help in regulating the excruciating pain. Though these drugs like any other medication need to be used in moderation. If not it will affect the functioning of your liver and function. Therefore ensure that these drugs are not being used for a long period of time, especially when you consume alcohol on a regular basis.

- **Clinical trials**

Almost all of the research centers and pharmaceutical companies, all over the world conduct clinical trials. Clinical trial is the process adopted by these institutions to test the viability of a new drug. The results of a clinical trial can go either ways. Therefore it is a chance that the individual will have to take and the outcome can be in his favor or not. But this is an option which can be considered when none o of the existing treatments seem to prove effective. But before you enroll yourself in any of the clinical trials, consult your doctor and you can also look into the support groups to help you get a better understanding of this concept.

- **Medical Treatments**

There are several medical treatments that will help you deal with the symptoms o peripheral neuropathy. Like I Have stated earlier, the treatment adopted will depend upon the area and the nerve affected, the type of treatment will also depend upon the underlying cause of the condition. There are some treatments, which have been discussed in this chapter.

Blood transfusion is considered to be a good option. In blood transfusion your body is drained of the blood present in your body and the same is replaced by blood from a different source. Plasmpherisis is a type of blood transfusion and what this does is it helps in removing the antibodies that have the potential to cause irritation to the patient. And such antibodies are removed from the individual's blood stream. A nerve block is also considered to be a good option. In a nerve block, a certain quantity of anesthetic will be injected into the nerves directly. Thereby numbing the pain. TENS stands for transcutaneous electronic nerve stimulation; this is one method, which might not work for everyone. It is a drug free therapy, therefore many patients like to consider this option though it might or might not work. In Transcutaneous electronic nerve stimulation, there are electrodes, which are placed on an individual's skin, and then small amount so of electricity is transmitted into the skin. What this method does is, it reduces or disrupts the transmission of signals of pain from the brain to the sensory organs. Thereby reducing the pain felt by an individual. Another form of treatment, which can be considered, is the use of ergonomic casts; these ergonomic casts will help the affected areas of the individual's like hands, feet, legs or even arms. This cast provides the support required to ensure that the person's discomfort has been reduced. This is also method of pain reduction. The discomfort a person who suffers from carpal tunnel syndrome will be reduced with the use of the cast. This helps to keep the wrists in a position, which is convenient while sleeping.

All the above-mentioned treatments are helpful in reducing the pain experienced by a person who is suffering from peripheral neuropathy.

- **Self care**

Self-care is perhaps the easiest and the least intrusive of all the options available to a person suffering from peripheral neuropathy. In addition to the pain relives which can be bought over the counter, there have been many successful cases in which people suffering from peripheral neuropathy have found relief through different treatments such as chiropractic sessions and even acupuncture. Acupuncture is the process where tiny needles are inserted into the key areas of the body. Massage, meditation and yoga, which have been present since hundreds of years are considered to be very effective to deal with any problem faced by an individual and peripheral neuropathy is no exception. Like I have mentioned earlier, regular exercising can also help in reducing the discomfort faced by an individual. Cutting back on smoking and alcohol, if you consume either of these regularly then reducing or altogether stopping these will prove helpful. Because these habits will do nothing apart from increasing the nerve damage sustained and will just deteriorate your condition. So please stay away from these two, if you want to reduce your own suffering.

- ***Make Your Home Safe***

Peripheral neuropathy is one such condition wherein the messages transmitted from your brain and spinal cord to all the other parts of your body is disrupted. Therefore this results in making you either overly sensitive or even completely insensitive towards pain or any other sensations. If you are suffering from peripheral neuropathy, then it is a very good idea to make your home safe for yourself. Because the risk of such people suspecting to accidents at home is greater than it is for the rest. Your feet are especially more vulnerable or prone to accidents. Therefore ensure that you always wear shoes or footwear of some sort to protect your feet. Keep your floor clean and get rid of all those objects that might cause you to trip and fall. Taking this precaution will reduce your likelihood of experiencing a fall. In peripheral neuropathy the sensations in your hands and feet will be affected. To make sure that you don't burn yourself while using water to clean the dishes or even bathe, check the temperature of the water using your elbow and not your hands and feet. To prevent any further accidents, install antislip bath mats and handrails in your bathroom. Because slipping and falling on a wet floor is one of the most common causes of enduring nerve damage. Sitting or remaining in one position for a long duration of time will also affect your nerves. So, do not sit in one position for too long. Move around for a couple of minutes after every hour. Those who have work that involves or requires them to sit down for long duration of time should consider this seriously.

- ***Therapy***

There are various therapies and procedures, which will prove beneficial in reducing the symptoms you, might exhibit from peripheral neuropathy. Physical therapy is a very good option if you have weakness in your muscles. Physical therapy will not just help in reducing this weakness but it will also help in improving your movements. Ease of movements is always a positive sign. Using different forms of support like leg braces, a walking stick, wheelchair or even a cane will facilitate in better movement and provide your body with the required physical activity without causing much discomfort to the individual. Treatments that involve the exchange of plasma and also the infusion of intravenous immunoglobulin will help in reducing the symptoms shown by a person suffering from peripheral neuropathy. People who have some underlying inflammatory conditions will definitely benefit from these activities and it will also help in reducing the hyperactivity of the immune system that makes it attack its own self. In plasma exchange, the blood form the patients' body is removed and thereby getting rid of the unnecessary antibodies and proteins from your blood. And then once again putting this refined blood into the person's body once again. In immune globulin therapy the exact opposite of the previous procedure is done. Instead of removing antibodies from blood, the patient's blood will be infused with high levels of a particular protein, which will work as antibodies. These methods are considered to be intrusive. And like I have mentioned earlier the process of TENS is less intrusive and is drug free therapy. In Transcutaneous electrical nerve stimulation gentle bolts of electricity are generated into the person's skin to disrupt the signals of pain. Good results can be seen if this therapy is followed for a month with a session each day for 30 minutes. The cause of peripheral neuropathy can also be increased pressure on nerves and this pressure can be caused due to the presence of tumors or any leisions. The best way to get rid of such tumors is by surgery. This will not only ensure the removal f tumors but it will also ensure that the pressure on these nerves has been relieved, thereby reducing the pain experienced by a person.

All the above-mentioned treatments will help in reducing the signs and symptoms displayed by a person who is suffering from peripheral neuropathy.

Over-the-counter Medications for Diabetic Peripheral Neuropathy

Early stages of diabetic neuropathy are comparatively easier as the pain isn't severe. Over-the-counter medications may be adequate to relieve pain. However, as the disease progresses, over the counter medications are not enough. Here are some of the most prescribed types of medicine.

Acetaminophen is a group of painkillers. It is an analgesic. Tylenol for instance is an acetaminophen, and it works by blocking nerves from transmitting signals of pain to the brain. Acetaminophen makes it harder for the sensation of pain to travel via the nerves to the brain, rendering the brain and thus our bodies to feel the pain. Possible side effects: liver damage (if taken for a long time).

Non-steroidal anti-inflammatory drugs or NSAIDs have a two-fold effect—they fight inflammation and also work as painkillers. They block the body from producing 'prostaglandins' or chemicals that cause inflammation and pain. By ingesting NSAID, you suppress prostaglandins, thus easing inflammation and pain. Some common over-the-counter NSAIDs are Motrin, Advil, and Aleve.
Possible side effects: stomach ulcers, diarrhea, nausea, and fatigue.

Topical Medications are those that you directly apply to your skin. The most commonly used one for diabetic peripheral neuropathy patients is capsaicin cream. Capsaicin is the chemical that makes chilli peppers hot, and it does relieve pain as well. It is just a temporary measure, and thus you'll need to apply at regular intervals. Topical medications are generally used for foot pain.

Prescription Medicines for Diabetic Peripheral Neuropathy

Quite often, people with peripheral diabetic nerve pain need specifically prescribed medications to treat the pain, as they are stronger. Very often, combinations of these medicines are required to deal with the various effects of nerve damage. FDA has approved two medicines for diabetic peripheral neuropathy: Lyrica and Cymbalta. Speak to you doctor and find out if these medications may be the ones suitable for your treatment. Of course, there are many more medications available to treat diabetic neuropathy. Side effects of most of these medicines are headache, insomnia, and nausea

Anti-depressants are one of the mainstays for treatment of diabetic neuropathy:

Tricyclic anti-depressants act by raising levels of neurotransmitters that calm your brain, and also can reduce pain. They also lift your mood and help you sleep (sleeping either severe nerve pain is difficult). For nerve pain due to diabetes, amitriptyline (for instance, Tryptano and Elavil), desipramine (for instance, Pertofrane and Norpramin), and imipramine (like Deprinol and Antideprin) are usually prescribed. Referred to as 'first line' medications because they are among the first few medications doctors usually prescribe for neuropathy relief. They are effective and safe as well. Side effects may include drowsiness, dizziness, dry mouth, dry eyes, and constipation as well.

Serotonin-norepinephrine reuptake inhibitors (SNRIs), usually called SNRIs, increase serotonin and norepinephrine in your system by blocking them from being reabsorbed by your brain. Increased serotonin and norepinephrine levels improve mental balance and reduce pain. Commonly prescribed to treat diabetic neuropathy, it is FDA-approved for the same. Side effects like drowsiness, dizziness, and insomnia may appear.

Selective serotonin reuptake inhibitors or SSRIs increase the levels of serotonin in your system. They block serotonin reuptake to increase the serotonin level in your body. More serotonin, means less pain perception. Some examples: citalopram (Celexa) and paroxetine (Paxil).

Anti-seizure medications, also called anti-convulsants or anti-epileptics are used to treat seizures. They work by slowing down nerve signals in patients with diabetic neuropathy and reduce pain effectively. Some prominent anti-seizures and anti-convulsants medications are gabapentin (Neurontin and Gabarone) and Pregabalin (Lyrica). FDA has approved Lyrica for treatment of diabetic peripheral neuropathy. Side effects are weight gain, drowsiness, nausea and dizziness.

Opioids (also called Narcotics) are one the most extreme heavy-duty painkillers. They help provide fast and stable relief from severe pain, but can be addictive as well. So, one must be very careful when using these. These can only be done under specific advice (and a prescription) from a trained doctor.
Tramadol (examples: Ultram or Ultracet) and Oxycodone (OxyContin) have proven to be best suited to relieving pain due to diabetic neuropathy.
Possible side effects with opioids include drowsiness, nausea, and constipation.

Topical Medication like capsaicin cream, are usually available without any prescriptions. A great topical medication is called lidocaine patch. However, you must have a prescription to purchase a lidocaine patch. An example of a lidocaine patch is Lidoderm.

Important: Please keep in mind that diabetic peripheral neuropathy also gives rise to a host of other conditions, like urinary tract infection or other digestive problems that happen in patients of autonomic neuropathy. To treat these conditions, we may often need to take other medicines as prescribed by a doctor.

Manage peripheral neuropathy

It is essential for the person who is suffering from peripheral neuropathy to be able to manage this condition. Here are some steps that you can take that will help manage peripheral neuropathy.

- It is extremely important to take care of your feet. And the stress on this point becomes exponentially high if you are suffering from diabetes. Check your feet daily for bruises, cuts, calluses or even lesions. Wearing cotton socks which are lose and airy along with soft soled shoes will help. If your feet are extremely sensitive, then purchasing a semicircular hoop which is available at any local medical supply store will be a good investment.
- Exercising is important. Period. Whatever you age might be, a little bit of exercise will go a long way. But before you jump into a rigorous mode of exercising, consult your doctor and move. Exercise in the form of walking thrice a week will help improve the blood pressure, increase the strength of your muscles and also control the blood sugar level. There are other options o f exercising such as yoga and tai chi.
- Smoking kills. It literally does. If you are suffering from peripheral neuropathy, it will do you some good if you quit smoking. Because smoking has been proved to increase the risk of foot problems and also cause other neuropathic conditions.
- Eating right is extremely helpful. Healthy eating habits are essential to maintain proper metabolism of your body. Meals which are low in fat and high in vitamins, proteins and other nutrients will help in managing the peripheral neuropathy.
- Excessive alcohol needs to cut down on and stopping the

consumption of alcohol altogether is an extremely good idea.
- Also keep a close check on your glucose levels. If you have diabetes, your blood sugar levels can go berserk without a moment's notice.

CHAPTER 6: PREVENTION OF PERIPHERAL NEUROPATHY

Peripheral neuropathy is an extremely difficult disorder to deal with. Like the old saying goes "prevention is better than cure" there are certain steps that you can take to avoid contracting peripheral neuropathy. It is always to avoid something, especially when you have the power to do s instead of having to live with the consequences. The following tips will aid you in avoiding peripheral neuropathy:

- **Managing the underlying conditions**

There is always an underlying condition, which is responsible for causing peripheral neuropathy. Therefore the best way to deal with peripheral neuropathy is by managing the underlying condition or the cause for it. These conditions can vary from exposure to toxins, alcoholism, diabetes, or even rheumatoid arthritis.

- **Healthy lifestyle**

A healthy lifestyle will always have a positive effect on your health. And this is one thing that is in your indisputable control. Therefore if you make choices that are healthy then you will be able to prevent peripheral neuropathy. And lifestyle choices can vary from selecting a healthy diet to the way you exercise and live. Let us take a look at some examples so that you can get a better understanding of this:

- Try consuming a diet which is well balanced and healthy, with all the nutrients your body will require to function normally. A diet which is rich in vegetables, fruits, whole grains and lean protein is always helpful in keeping your nerves healthy. B-12 is one of the most common deficiencies faced by many. You will need to consume meats, fish, eggs, dairy products low in fat and fortified cereals to help protect against this deficiency. If you are a non-vegetarian, there are many meats that you can regularly consume to avoid this deficiency. But if you are a vegetarian or a vegan, then you need to consume fortified cereal because these are rich in B-12. Consult your doctor or nutritionist to devise a dietary plan that will keep your body healthy and thoroughly nourished. Even consuming B-12 supplements is a very good option.

- Exercising regularly has proven to make individuals lead a healthier life. If you aren't sure about how to go about it, then consult your doctor. With the doctor's consent you can start exercising at least three times a day. The sessions need not be tiring or excruciating. Even a brisk walk will do. So start exercising at least three times a day for 30 minutes each, you will definitely see improvement.
- One of the easiest things you can do is to avoid those factors which are likely to cause damage to your nerves. Nerve damage might be caused due to excess stress over the muscles and also due to repetitive movements, exposure to toxins, alcoholism, smoking or even sitting in cramped positions.
- If peripheral neuropathy is present in your family's history then you can prevent this disorder from occurring by eating a healthier diet, exercising moderately, avoiding smoking or even quitting it and the same applies to alcohol too.
- If you know the kind of toxins you might be exposed to at your work or anywhere else, taking certain precautions to protect yourself is a good idea. While playing sports, always keep your feet covered, especially when the sport concerned involves kicking. And lastly by never inhaling toxic substances such as glue to get high will help you reduce the risk of contracting peripheral neuropathy.

If you are suffering from diabetes, it is essential that you take good care of your feet. You will need to wash, clean and inspect your feet daily and even constantly moisturizing to keep your skin moist will help greatly. These simple steps will help you prevent the onset of peripheral neuropathy. The above-mentioned tips weren't difficult and in fact are totally doable.

CHAPTER 7: ALTERNATIVE TREATMENTS

Some people with DPN surprisingly find relief in relatively simple ways. Sometimes it may be a simple warm or cold bath, and sometimes a session of acupuncture.

Alternative medicine

We have already looked at all the medicine related treatments available for dealing with peripheral neuropathy. People who are suffering from peripheral neuropathy look into other forms of complementary and alternative therapies, which will help absolve them of pain from their symptoms. These therapies have proved to be effective in certain cases, though there isn't any strong research to prove this point. Now let us look at some alternative medicines available:

- One form of alternative therapy is acupuncture. In acupuncture thin needles are inserted into a person's body at different points and it may help in reducing the symptoms of peripheral neuropathy. Though you will need to sit through multiple sessions to notice any improvement in your condition. Ensure that you get acupuncture done from a professional and also make sure that the needles used are sterile, to avoid contracting any infections.
- Alpha lipoic acid is an antioxidant and this has been used for treating peripheral neuropathy for years in Europe. But before you go ahead with this therapy ensure that you have consulted your doctor about its use. Because, this antioxidant can interfere with the levels of blood sugar and has some side effects too. The side effects include a skin rash and an upset stomach.
- Primrose oil and certain other herbs have the ability to help in reducing the pain suffered by such individuals who are suffering from neuropathy. But before you go ahead with this treatment too, consult your doctor. Do not forget to consult your doctor about whatever alternate therapy that you would like to try.
- Amino acids can also help in improving this disorder in those people who have undergone chemotherapy and also in people who are suffering from diabetes. Thought there are certain side effects like nausea and vomiting.

- Fish oils contain omegs3 fatty acids and these will reduce inflammation and also improve the blood flow. This will help in improving the condition of neuropathy in diabetic individuals. But do consult your doctor before you start taking supplements made of fish oil if you are on any anti clogging medicines.

Alpha lipoic acid or ALA

An antioxidant called alpha lipoic acid (or ALA) and can be taken as a pill form, provided effective relief from pain in people with diabetic neuropathy. ALA has already been proved to reduce pain and numbness in diabetic neuropathy patients. Also called thioctic acid, it clears free radicals from your body, thus reducing nerve damage.

ALA has been extremely effective in treating DPN, however the side effects of treatment—vomiting, nausea and dizziness—increase with the dosage. It has been seen a dose of 600 milligrams once daily appeared to be the most effective.

ALA is made in small amounts by our body but is not found in any food we eat. It contains lots of sulphur. It also works as an antioxidant and not only helps protect against pain arising out of DPN, but may also aids in production and functioning of insulin, improves blood circulation, and decrease oxidative stress in people with diabetes. Antioxidants also help keep you young and rejuvenate all your body organs from inside out!

It is important to discuss taking ALA therapy with your doctor before you start. ALA has been known to increase the risk of hypoglycemia (low blood glucose) in patients who inject insulin or use certain diabetes drugs. It possibly interferes with absorption of the vitamin biotin as well. Remember that the U.S. Food and Drug Administration (FDA) do not regulate ALA supplements, like other food supplements, for effectiveness, quality and side effects.

Preventing Neuropathic Pain with Foot Care

Nerve pain due to DPN may take you to a doctor, but the numbness arising out of DPN can take you straightaway to the hospital. Numbness tends to make our foot devoid of any sensations. Consequently, when our foot gets burnt, or badly cut or hurt in any way, we do not even notice it and leave them untreated. Complications may lead to festering infections, poorly healing ulcers and even amputations.

Suggested foot care:

Inspect and clean them every day. Any ulcer or sore that isn't healing as fast as it requires a visit to a podiatrist.

Comfortable shoes are a must. There are stores that specialize in shoes for neuropathic feet. You can specially order shoes that suit you best.

Wear padded socks that protect your toes and the heel.

Visit a podiatrist regularly. An average podiatrist might charge you $10, but considering the risks, the money spent is definitely worth it, and more so if your foot is in critical condition.

Vitamin B Complex May Help Nerve Pain

Vitamin B, (in its many forms like B-1, B-12, B-6, and folic acid) is essential for maintenance of your nerve health. Most people get enough B vitamins just from eating a healthy diet

They are generally inexpensive, and absolutely safe and help some people. Suggest amounts for intake are:

25 mg of thiamine (B-1),

500 micrograms of B-12,

25 milligrams of B-6, and

At least 1 milligram of folic acid.

Precautions: higher doses of B-6 can lead to toxicity, pain and numbness in your hands and legs, and in extreme cases, you may even face difficulty walking.

Evening Primrose Oil and Diabetic Neuropathy

Evening primrose oil is extracted from the evening primrose plant and is rich in omega-6 fatty acids that are important structural components of cell walls. Theoretically, evening primrose oil, which is also available in pills, may aid in repair of damaged nerves cells or help them regenerate.

In certain tests, ingesting evening primrose oil orally somewhat improved nerve function in people with DPN. The risks of taking evening primrose oil are relatively minor in most, but people who take daily aspirin or prescription blood thinners (anticoagulants) are more at risk (it may lead to bleeding) and these patients are advised to get it ratified by their doctors first.

Multiple capsules may be needed and to find out exactly how much you need, a visit to your doctor is essential.

Biofeedback for Diabetes Neuropathy

It is possible to train the body to decrease the severity of diabetes nerve pain through biofeedback. The trick is to try consciously controlling a body function that is otherwise regulated by the body and there are ways to control things like skin temperature, blood pressure or heart rate.

Sounds like science fiction? It happens! There has been quite a lot of positive evidence about the benefits of biofeedback. Already, it has been used to help control epilepsy seizures, migraine pain, high blood pressure, and some other functions.

Here is how it works. You have to wear sensors on your head or elsewhere depending on what you are attempting to control. These sensors let you "hear", "see" or "feel" certain functions like digestion, pulse, muscle tension and body temperature. The dancing lines and beeps on monitors you can see reflect what's going on inside your body. Gradually you are assisted till you learn to control those squiggles and beeps. A few sessions later, you would be surprised to realize that your mind has trained your biological system and you can exert substantial control. According to experts and practitioners say that it is not a hard thing to master!

Meditation to Relieve Diabetes Nerve Pain

Meditation is offered as a therapy in various pain treatment centers around the world for diabetes (and related conditions like DPN) and other painful disorders as well. Research has also shown that meditation can help one lower his/her blood pressure and also control breathing, heart rate and one's brain waves too! Tension and tightness from our muscles is released as our body gradually relaxes.

Repetition and focus is at the heart of meditation. Sit down and focus on your breath, ignore any external thoughts and keep repeating a word or phrase or anything that makes relaxes you. Various people have described feeling calm, warmth, and some even reported a sense of heaviness while meditating. You can visit a class. A few sessions will help you get into the thick of things.

Relaxation Techniques to Relieve Neuropathy Pain

Stress makes DPN pain worse. It is important that you learn to relax. One's breathing pattern may be affected by changes in one's emotions. That explains why managing your breathing is important to relaxation. Getting familiar with your own breathing pattern scan help you control stress level and pain as well. Most importantly, find a suitable location, a good state of mind and a comfortable body position. Try blocking out worries and thoughts that may distract you.

Relaxation techniques to help with diabetes nerve pain include:

Rhythmic breathing: Take slow, long breaths. Inhale and later exhale slowly. Slowly, count till five as you inhale do the same as you exhale. Paying attention to how your body tends to relax. That helps you relax better.

Deep breathing: breathing in an out slowly, till you can count up to 10 (slowly) or more if you can.

Visualized breathing: It is all about visualizing the breath coming into your lungs via your nostrils. Picture your expanding chest and contracting abdomen. Visualize exhaling the same way. Make yourself believe that you are slowly distressing yourself with each breath.

Relax to music: This one really needs no explanation.

Mental imagery (guided imagery) relaxation: A method of relaxation by imagining any imagery that soothes you. Simply daydream about having achieved what you really want to in life. It would give you a lot of pleasure.

CHAPTER 8: EFFECT OF NEUROPATHY ON YOUR LIFE

We have looked at what neuropathy means, the types of neuropathies, which are present, the causes of it, symptoms, and methods to prevent it and also alternative treatments available. But there is one more important area, which we still have not covered. And this aspect is the effect neuropathy will have y=on your life. Like with any other disorder, even peripheral neuropathy will have a negative impact on your life. The pain caused by neuropathy can have an overpowering affect on your day-to-day activities and the quality of your life in general. The symptoms exhibited by neuropathy can vary from being severe to extremely mild. The experiences of all those people who have suffered from neuropathy will be different. Though, if it has been identified at the appropriate stage and proper treatment is available, then the effects of neuropathy can be reduced or even controlled.

If you are suffering from neuropathy then you will experience excruciating pain, numbness, you will find it extremely difficult to stand for a long duration of time or even walk without any assistance, your sense of equilibrium will be affected and with this the risk of you falling will also increase, performing basic functions like buttoning your shirt or even tying your shoe laces might seem quite challenging, increased sensitivity towards heat or cold and also the lack of sensations. These are the whole gamut of symptoms any individual suffering from neuropathy is likely to experience and the effect these would have on the individual's life will be extremely negative. Not being able to perform the most basic of functions will be extremely hard for a person on a psychological and physical level.

Survivors of neuropathy need to stay away from extreme temperatures and always make use of protective clothing, because of their sensitivity towards temperature. If there is any numbness or insensitivity, then it is necessary that you take additional care and also that you pay attention towards the skin on your hands and feet, because you might have endured some wound and not even realize it.

If you experience any pain while going on with you day to day activities like wearing your shoes or even using the covers over your feet during the night, even this might seem difficult. There are many treatments, which are available for you to take into consideration that can help reduce the pain caused by these symptoms. Talk to your team of health care experts and also enquire about all the potential treatments available. Do not exclude or adopt any one treatment without talking to your doctor. If neuropathy affects your ability to drive a car, because it would affect the sensations in your feet then you should really not drive and should also consider a car, which is adapted for using hand controls. Insensitivity will make your reactions incredibly slow and might also cause an accident. This will not just increase your risk for being involved in an accident but it will also increase the risk faced by others.

Ask your health care provider to give you suggestions about the different steps which you can take and also the special equipment which will help you make your daily tasks easier. Consider exercising and even therapy sessions will prove to be beneficial. Safety measures will reduce your risk of accidentally hurting yourself. Joining a support group will prove to be helpful. Because for some neuropathy brings mental stress along with physical pain. Keep an eye out for signs, which might indicate depression, and when you notice any such symptoms, consult your doctor as soon as possible. With help from yourself and others will help you deal with neuropathy in a much better way.